Hypnosis sessions for deep sleep

Learn The Art Of Hpnosis Through The Collection Of The Best Hypnosis Sessions To Help Anyone To Sleep Deep

Melanie Johnson

Melanie Johnson

Melanie Johnson

© Copyright 2020 - All rights reserved.

Table of Contents

Melanie Johnson

Hypnosis for Deep Sleep

Welcome to a deep sleep session. I am going to assume that you are lying in the comfort of your own bed or someone else's bed. Please cover yourself up with a comfortable duvet if you are cold or lay on top the duvet if you are getting hot. Fluff your pillow before we begin because I want you to start in the most comfortable position possible.

Switch the light off and become aware of the background music in this session. Isn't it soothing? Allow your thoughts to flow with the calm rhythm of the sound you hear. As you fade the sound of the music just slightly, you grab onto the sound of my voice. Listen to the sound of my voice and the background music in harmonious balance. I want you to close your eyes. Your eyes are feeling droopy now. You have had a long day and your eyes are allowed to feel heavy. Keep your eyes closed and use your sense of hearing to follow my suggestions. You feel a deepening trust in my instructions with every word I speak. Allow my suggestions to flow through your mind, bringing more comfort with each moment.

You are going to focus on your breathing now. I want gentle inhales and exhales. Keep a consistent rhythm with each breath you take. Feel your body soften further with each exhale. Stop thinking about the thing that just crossed your mind and come back to me. I want you to feel a small wave of guilt for allowing your mind to wander. Now start your breathing over again. Small, shallow breaths—gently in and gently out. Keep doing this till you maintain an even rhythm. Allow your breathing to slow your heartbeat, one breath at a time. Your eyes are feeling more and drowsier with each beat of your heart. However, something is keeping your mind from giving into your fatigue. Your mind refuses to shut down and you don't know why. Shift your focus back to your breathing now and follow the air as it flows into your body. You can feel your body rise and fall as you inhale and follow the flow of air as it exits your body. You are becoming more confident in this session.

I want you to focus on your surroundings once your breathing is even and relaxed. What do you see? You only see darkness but this darkness seems to beckon you. There is a strange comfort in it. I want you to focus harder this time. Listen to your body inhaling and exhaling as you lay there. Indeed, there is something appearing in the darkness. What is it? It's just a little white speck.

Now I want you to focus on your body. Think about the way your head feels. Does it feel heavy? Strain your muscles a little and hold them for a moment. Feel the tension release from your muscles as you slowly relax them. Now your head feels clearer and more comfortable. Do the same with your neck. Make your muscles tense in your neck and hold for a moment. Count to three in your mind and then you may release them. Can you feel the tension of the day dissipate? All the horrible stress leaving your neck area. You feel more relaxed now.

Bring your focus back to the darkness for a moment before we continue. What do you see now? Oh, the white speck looks like a light, a very distant light. Can you hear any sounds yet? No? I didn't think so.

Shift your focus back to your body and pay attention to your arms this time. I want you to make tight fists with your hands and hold them. Now you can count to three again before you unclench your fists slowly. Allow yourself to become aware of the sensation of your action. Focus on the negative energy that is leaving your hands. Your arms feel relaxed now.

Go back to the darkness now. What do you see? The light has come closer now. Oh but wait, you can hear a distant sound now too. I want you to focus on that sound for a moment. You feel excited to find out what the sound is but with much focus, you still can't identify the sound.

Okay, come back to me again. I want you to pay attention to your stomach muscles now. Pull your stomach muscles and hold them for a moment. Keep holding them. Count to five this time and release. Focus on the comfort and relaxation the release has brought you. You are reaching a level of comfort that is strange to you. Welcome this newfound comfort.

Please go back to the darkness. I need you to know that I am here with you every moment of this session. Don't be afraid of anything. What do you see? The light has drawn nearer again. It's bright now and you can't quite make out what it is. Hear my voice speak calmness over you as the light approaches. The sound is getting louder now too but it's a disturbing sound. It would normally make you worry. However, you are not worried right now. You feel a deep-seated sense of safety in this session. Even though this feels strange and familiar at the same time, you know you must have been here before. You are finding it easier to overpower the sound with the calming background music now. Keep your focus on the music and the sound of my voice.

Let's return to your body once more. I want you to shift your attention to your legs. If you are not too far into your relaxation, I want you to move your ankles from side to side for a moment. Count to three and stop. Now you may pull your muscles stiff. Please don't strain them enough to injure yourself. Hold them like that for three seconds before releasing them. Pay close attention to how soft your legs feel now. You are in a deep state of relaxation, a state of mindfulness.

Now I want you to focus on your breathing again. Make sure it remains steady. Feel your body conform to each inhale and exhale. Your arms are too relaxed and you don't feel the need to touch your body to feel this. You are in an unfamiliar state of mind now. You have become one with your subconscious mind. You feel a deeper need to trust the sound of my voice now as the time draws nearer. All doubts have swiftly removed themselves. It's just you and my voice now.

Follow me back to the darkness that you have been curious about. There is a certain level of calm in this darkness. As it comes back into your inner sight, you see exactly what the light is. As a matter of fact, the sound is clear and distinct now. You are blinded by the light heading straight at you and deafened by the screeching noise. My voice is never silenced by this unbearable noise coming closer to you. The sound of metal grinding against metal makes you shift your attention to where you are standing. The bright light shows you the tracks beneath your feet. Your mind wanders off to an old western movie you've seen where someone looked like a deer stuck in headlights. Please bring your concentration back now. You feel your heart skip a beat for just a split second when suddenly, a great sense of calmness comes over you. You feel safe and accepting of this huge metal train coming your way. You are fully capable of stopping it dead in its tracks.

This train is filled with memories that plague your sleep every night. It's also filled with worries about tomorrow, the stresses of today and, various other thoughts and feelings. This is your own speeding train of thoughts that disrupts your sleep every night. A monstrous metal machine that won't leave you alone. This train comes to take away your peaceful darkness every night after you reach the first stage of sleep. It's a menace that makes you sit up for hours, fighting your heavy eyelids. The sound of this train alone is enough to drive anyone mad. It's the first time you are facing it directly, identifying it, and visualizing it.

Now I want you to concentrate hard on the background music and the sound of my voice. Keep your breathing steady and use welcomed sounds to drown the noise out. You know you can do it. Breathe in gently and breathe out slowly, one breath at a time. Listen to the calm tone of my voice and allow it to reassure your comfort and safety. Nothing will happen to you because you are stronger than you think. You know that this train is nothing more than a figment of your imagination. You also know that all those worries in the cargo can be dealt with tomorrow. There is no need to face this train now. Tomorrow is another day and trains shouldn't be running this late. You know your thoughts will be clearer when tomorrow comes.

Now listen closely to my suggestion. Allow every word to resonate through your mind. You have created this train; you have brought the image to life. Only you have the power to erase this image. Your imagination has brought it to life and your imagination will remove it. Now take your attention back to your breathing and focus on your heartbeat. Can you feel the steady rhythm of every beat? Take a moment and count your beats. Follow each beat and feel how it pumps the calmness through your veins. Now I know you are ready.

You stand on the train tracks, facing the oncoming train and know that you are now in control. You can control the trains every movement. You make the train slow down as you watch the sparks on the tracks from the train's brakes. The sound doesn't even penetrate your hearing anymore because you have drowned the sound out now. You can feel the vibrations in the tracks as the train draws nearer but you have no fear. You cannot fear something that doesn't exist in a physical form. You dig deep in your subconscious and find the strength you need to make this train vanish.

Suddenly, you are transported back into complete darkness. A darkness that feels safe and peaceful. You have successfully stopped the train and you're alone now. No thoughts or worries can cross your path anymore. Your physical form is feeling feather light now. You are connected to it and don't need to leave your darkness anymore. You feel proud of yourself and you have never felt this tired before. Your mind is still connected with your subconscious mind. Give your subconscious mind permission to leave you now. You will be perfectly fine in this quiet space. There are no more possible disruptions. You can feel yourself floating into a deeper, more peaceful state of sleep.

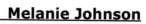

Melanie Johnson

Melanie Johnson

Deep Sleep Hypnosis Session

Now, I want you to get comfortable. Because you are trying to achieve a deep sleep, you should be lying down, your head resting on your most comfortable pillow and you are warmed by your softest blanket. Lie back and let your shoulders go slack, relaxing against the cushion of your bed. Gently close your eyes and release all the tension from your muscles. Release the tension in your arms, then your legs. Let go of the tension in your chest and in your back. All of the muscles in your body begin to feel looser and looser and your body is feeling light.

Focus your attention on your toes. Softly wiggle all ten toes once, and then again. Feel the energy released from your movement and the stillness that follows. Your toes are now ready for sleep.

Next, tighten the muscles in your calves and hold for one, two, three seconds. Now release the muscles.

Tighten them again for one, two, three seconds. Now release. The excess energy that keeps you up at night has been expelled from your calves. Your calves are now ready for sleep.

Next, squeeze your thigh muscles and hold for one, two, three seconds. Now release. The tension that was once stored there has been released. Your thighs are now ready for sleep. Feel the lightness that has cloaked your legs. Your legs feel weightless as if they could float up to the ceiling.

Focus your attention on your buttocks. Tighten your muscles in buttocks for one, two, three seconds. Now release the muscles. The tightness in your buttocks and lower back has been relieved. Your buttocks and lower back are now ready for sleep.

Focus your attention on your abdomen. Squeeze your abdominal muscles for one, two, three seconds. Now release. The anxiety that has been stored up and deterring sleep has been released. Your abdomen is now ready for sleep.

Concentrate on your chest. Tighten the muscles in your chest for one, two, three seconds. Now release. The sadness that has been weighing on you and preventing your mind from resting has been expelled. Your chest is now ready for sleep.

Direct your attention now to your shoulders. Tighten the muscles in your shoulder for one, two, three seconds. Now release. The stress that has been building in the deep tissue of your shoulders has now been dissolved. Your shoulders are now ready for sleep.

Focus your attention on your neck. Gently tighten the muscles and hold for one, two, three seconds. Now release. Gently tighten the muscles in your jaw and hold for one, two, three seconds. Now release. Gently tighten the muscles in your mouth and hold for one, two, three seconds. Now release. Gently squeeze your eyelids tighter for one, two, three seconds. Now release. The tension that was held in your face has now been released.

The entirety of your body has been washed with serenity as you expel the negative energy from your muscles. Now that your body is relaxed, your mind can now relax in preparation for deep slumber. Realize how free it feels to let go of all built up tension. In this moment nothing else matters. You are free. You are relaxed. You are weightless.

There is nowhere for you to be and you have everything you need. You are here, in this moment, permitting the calming sensation to course through your body. Your thoughts drift away. You don't try to follow or catch them. With each breath you take, you are feeling more and more serene. Breathe in, welcoming peace and harmony to your soul. Breathe out, exhaling all the negative energy and releasing your control. Realize how good it feels to be so relaxed.

Focus on being as relaxed as you can be at this moment. Allow your mind to settle down a little, to quiet, to be still. Instead, focus more on your body. How does it feel lying in your bed? Examine the coziness you feel beneath your sheets. Feel how smooth your sheets are and gentle weight of your blanket on top of you. Relax in the embrace of the softest bed in the world. You are content in every way.

Imagine that on the other side of the room is an open fire crackling. The orange and yellow flames emanate a sensation of calmness as its soft light can be seen upon your walls and ceiling. You feel the warmth of this sensation. You watch closely as the flames flicker and dance upon the logs. The sound of the crackling fire reminds you that you are safe in this space. In this bed you are warm, cozy, and protected.

Scan your body for tension. Find where you still hold stress in your body. Examine your shoulders, your neck, your temples, and your back. Find the stress that is hiding and release it. Allow your body to feel relieved, relaxed, at peace.

Examine the aroma of the fire as it fills the room. The fragrance is deep and musky. It reminds you of good memories with the ones who love you. These memories remind you that your life is beautiful. Place both hands on your stomach, one below your ribs and one above your belly button. Take a deep breath in through your nose, inhale those good memories. Let the air fill your belly and your hands rise on top of your abdomen. Then, through your nose, exhale all of the negativity you have collected. The worries that you harbor are no longer welcome here.

Breathe in the relaxing scent of the fireplace; fill up your stomach like it is a balloon. Let your hands move as your inhale. Then exhale any remaining tension. You now feel loose and at ease. There is calmness that envelope your body as you breathes. As you feel more relaxed, you hear only the fire in this quiet space. The quietness of the room also quiets your mind and you welcome rest and relaxation.

As you lay, keep breathing and reveling in this blissful setting: you're tucked inside your cozy bed with a fire to keep you warm. Focus on this serene moment and give yourself permission to enjoy it. Remember that you are in control. Many times, your mind is overthinking, overanalyzing, and too critical. In this moment, it is you who is in control and you will exhale those negative thoughts. As you exhale, you regain your balance and you feel content. Your body feels looser, lighter, and a weight is lifted off your chest.

Your body is light and warm as you listen to my voice. Let me guide you as you drift off. I'm going to count now and you will listen. Let my voice lull you. You are safe and relaxed and warm.

Ten... Your body is entirely loose and relaxed.

Nine... You are in a peaceful, calm, and safe environment.

Eight... You can feel the warmth and love of those who care about you, enveloping your senses.

Seven... The sound of the burning fire, the crackling of wood lulls you further into an even deeper state of relaxation.

Six... You inhale all of the good in the world with each breath you take.
Five... You exhale all the bad, expelling all of your stress and anxiety with each breath out.

Four... You feel your bodies getting lighter until you are almost like a feather in the breeze.

Three... You feel your mind becoming heavier and brimming with warmth and love.

Two... Accept the peace that has engulfed you, understand that it is good. Let it send you off ever deeper into the feeling of relaxation.

One... You feel yourself drifting all the way down, as deep as you can go, nearer to the bottom, towards warmth and sleep.

You are safe and you are relaxed. Allow yourself to feel safe and relaxed in this space.

Imagine that you are a leaf on a tree. You are connected to a giant colony of other leaves attached to a branch. That branch is attached to a trunk. You are a part of a busy, ever rustling tree.

However, you want to be still. You need to rest. You need to separate yourself from the busyness of your world. You decide that you will depart your branch and you begin to float. Slowly, as if gravity has slowed your fall, you twirl and roll in the breeze. You are peacefully drifting further and further, reassured that you are safe.

Instead of the ground, you see that there is a quiet pond below your tree and soon you will touch the surface. As you float towards it, you notice its stillness. There are no ripples or disturbances. The surface is smooth and clear; it is as reflective as a mirror. As you reach the water, you greet the surface with a delicate kiss.

You send gentle, peaceful ripples from your contact. Concentric circles echo out to the edges of the pond. This energy radiates from you until the last ripple falls away. It is now you on the water, undisturbed and immersed in the tranquility of your setting. You drift on the surface of your unconsciousness. You feel the warmth of the water beneath you and surrounding you. The water is so soothing that you feel yourself getting heavier. You feel as though you could keep floating deeper and deeper beneath the surface until you fell asleep.

The relaxation that you feel now is beckoning you closer to rest, to deep sleep. Notice how relaxed you are in this very moment. Notice how soothing the sensations are in your body. Breathe in the relaxation that the water provides. Breathe out any tension you have.

I am going to count down from five. When I reach one, you are going to fully embrace the peace that has engulfed you and lose yourself in sleep. You will feel yourself slipping into a calm and serene rest.

Five... You think of the still surface of the pond, and how it provided safety for you, the leaf. The calm water is summoning your sleep.

Four... You feel the warmth of tranquility ripple from the top of your scalp and down your neck. It glides through your shoulders, radiates through your chest and stomach, and finally glazes over your legs. You are encompassed by this sensation.

Three... You feel your body become heavy and you softly sink in a little deeper to your consciousness. You are safe and protected.

Two... You feel yourself drift away, like your leaf on the still pond. You float away, quietly into the night.

One... You are now asleep, resting and at peace.

Breathe in, breathe out. Breathe in, breathe out. When you wake up, you will be renewed and refreshed and ready to take on the day. You will be ready to conquer the obstacles of your life now that you have conquered sleep.

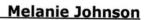 **Melanie Johnson**

Hypnosis for Overthinking Cure Session

Now I would love to guide you on an amazing trip and remove your habit of overthinking everything. Let me start by bringing your focus to my voice. Pay attention to the strong force drawing you to my voice as I speak. This force grows stronger with every word I say.

Find yourself a comfortable and quiet space to sit or lay down, either is good. Make sure you are undisturbed and open the windows to feel the fresh air. Bring your focus back to my voice and pay close attention to the sounds around you. The sound of relaxing music and my voice are the only two sounds you can hear now. I would love to use a method I once used on a friend for this session. My friend was filled with fear that stopped her from doing what she wanted. It caused her to overthink every possible task before jumping in.

Enough about that now. I want you to focus on your breathing as you lay or sit as comfortably as possible.

Take a deep inhalation in and keep it for a moment. Now release it slowly. Pay attention to the air as it crosses your lips and take note of how it feels. Can you feel the tension crossing your lips? Now I want you to think hard about a fear you have, a fear you face every day. One that has stopped you from doing something incredible. Now for the scary part. Take a deep breath, sucking in the air around you. Hold it for a moment. Just a little longer. Now force that air out. The air you inhaled was polluted by your fear. You have taken the first step to facing your fear.

Keep your thoughts with my voice as I help you relax your tense muscles now. Carry on taking deep but gentle breaths now and hold each one for just a moment. Exhale softly, without too much force this time. Don't stop doing this. I want you to listen inside. Can you hear it? Can you hear the racing beat of your heart? Allow the rapid beat of your heart to be second to the sound of my voice.

Melanie Johnson

I want you to start with your head. Tense your head by allowing anger to possess it. Hold this tension for a few seconds. One, two, and release slowly. Take note of the way your head feels now. The fear that was stored in your muscles has been crushed by your tension. Next, I want you to do the same with your neck and shoulders. Force your muscles into a tense position. Hold. One, two, and release. Notice how fearless they feel now.

Keep listening to my voice as I speak to you. Every word bringing you one step closer to relief. Move your focus to your arms and tense your muscles. Hold. One, two, and release. Listen to your racing heartbeat as your arms melt like jelly. You will repeat this exercise with your legs and feet next. Pull your legs into a straight and tense position and hold them like that.

One, two, and release. Pay close attention to the absence of fear in your legs. A wonderful sense of relaxation overcomes them. Shift your attention to your chest area while you allow my voice to keep you calm.

Feel your chest rise and fall with every breath you take, remembering to hold each breath for just a moment.

Listen to the rhythm of your heart. It's still racing but has slowed quite a bit now. Count every heartbeat until you get to ten. I will give you a moment to do this. Keep your breathing consistent throughout your counts. You can feel a calm effect traveling through your physical body. Your body is just melting into your bed or chair. I want you to breathe deeply and hold it. One, two, and release gently. Move your focus back to your heartbeat and count the beats again. One, two, three, four, five, six, seven, eight, nine, and ten.

I want you to bring your core focus back to my suggestion now and listen to every word. Feel safer with every word you hear. Allow your heartbeat to move back to a secondary sound. It's important to keep it in earshot throughout the session. Now I want you to bring your imagination into full focus. Allow my voice to carry your imagination into an alternate place. You trust me and every inch of you believes that you can follow me.

Start opening your mind's eye slowly, allowing your imagination to take over. An image is developing in front of your mind's eye as it opens. You look down and notice that you are wearing odd clothes, not your own clothes. You are wearing a red jumpsuit with bright yellow stripes down the side. You want to touch it with your hand but you are wearing gloves. You can feel the cold leather around your skin. You start feeling weight on your back that wasn't there before, a heavy weight. Your head also feels heavier because you appear to be wearing a helmet. You notice someone sitting across from you as your image comes into focus. You know this person because she is a close friend. You can't hear her but you see her mouth moving. She must be talking. She is all dressed in the same ridiculous get up as you. You can feel the roar of an engine beneath you. The roar is trying to penetrate your mind but I am still here. Your guide is with you all the way.

_____

There is a sudden gush of air that is deafening. You look to your right and there is a door that has been opened. The entire image is becoming clear now. You are on a small plane and have been suited up for a dive. Deep down inside you feel a small sense of calm despite your location.

My voice has become deeper and louder now, penetrating your subconscious mind and soothing your fears. You shift focus to your heartbeat as you breathe and hold. One, two and release. Keep your breathing calm at all times. Your heartbeat is faster than normal but not too fast.

Suddenly, your subconscious mind wanders off to think about all the possible outcomes; trying to analyze all the risks of what you're about to do. Stop! Breathe deep and hold. One, two, and release the air and the fear along with it.

You move closer to courage with every word I speak and every breath you take. You look down at your hands and see the tremors calm down, little by little.

You listen to your heartbeat as you glance across at your best friend and she smiles at you. It's a genuine smile that slows your heart down more. Thump thump thump. You feel relaxed enough to return the smile.

You can feel your fears leaving your body as your smile stretches across your face. Your friend is speaking to you but the noises are cancelling her voice out. You focus hard on the sound of my voice and the peaceful music in the background.

This takes your focus away from all the terrible noise and now you can start hearing your friend. She gets up and approaches you, telling you how proud she is that you have come with her.

You want to utter negativity as she takes your hand but you control your urge and allow her to take your hand.

You feel proud of yourself in this moment and you give her hand a reassuring squeeze.

Your friend asks if you're ready and you just nod in agreement as she gently pulls you up, never letting go of your hand. You feel relaxed with her touch and the sound of my voice guiding you.

All terrible thoughts have stopped racing through your mind. You have chosen one and that is the thought of enjoying the dive from a small plane in the middle of nowhere. Nothing will go wrong now.

You follow your friend closer to the door and she asks if you would like to keep holding hands. You nod in agreement again with a bigger smile this time.

Take a moment to listen to your heartbeat and the sound of my suggestions. Please be aware that your heart has stopped racing, it has slowed to a normal rhythm now.

Take a deep breath in again and hold it there for a moment. You feel good as you release it. You take a step forward while holding your friends hand and look out the door. You can see the amazing fields below with the ocean just a short distance to the right.

The gusts of wind no longer bother you. You cannot hear it anymore. You feel yourself take the final step forward while holding your friend's hand. You can feel her support in her touch.

You have the greatest sense of freedom as the two of you enter the freefall. You cannot describe the rush of positive emotions flowing through you.

You feel your friend's hand in yours and relax into a euphoric state.

You can feel your friend is in the same place. You are sharing an incredible experience with her.

_____

Melanie Johnson

An experience you would surely have missed if you allowed your fear to control your thoughts. My voice momentarily becomes secondary to the joy you feel. You are falling and the fresh air is rushing past your skin. You can feel the droplets from the sea around your face.

The sound becoming a faint whistle past your ears. Now I need you to come back to my voice and focus.

You use your free hand to pull the tag, releasing your parachute. There is a sudden tug when your parachute opens.

Your friend lets go of your hand and you watch her move away to open her own parachute. She never removes her calming smile from her face for a single moment.

This is the exact moment you realize you have conquered your fear and you have stopped thinking about all the things that could have gone wrong.

You have finally allowed yourself to be free and you know you can't control everything.

You pay close attention to my suggestions as you approach your landing field.

Continue breathing as you count backwards from ten. Ten, nine, eight, seven, six, five, four, three, two, and one.

You feel your feet gently touch the ground as you are whisked away from your imaginary image and back to your bed or chair. You can feel the comfort and safety of your physical presence again. I need you to be conscious of the smile you have naturally stretched on your face, a genuinely happy smile.

Take a deep breath. Hold it for a moment and release it gently. Listen to your heartbeat's perfect slow rhythm as you descend back into your own body.

Use your right hand and put it on your chest and inhale. Hold it for a moment before you exhale slowly.

Feel your body become heavier as you are relaxed into your bed or seat; your physical presence fully restored.

Now breathe, open your eyes and feel like a new person.

Affirmations for Positive Energy and Thinking

An affirmation is a positive statement that reminds you of critical thought. In this meditation below, we have listed a number of affirmations. These are written from a first-person perspective. You can either repeat them back after they are declared or let these thoughts flow into your mind as if they were your own.

We don't always realize just how often we repeat negative affirmations to ourselves. Rather than letting your mind continue to be filled with negativity, look for a way to turn your outlook around completely. You'll want to start to notice the negative things that you say to yourself. These might notice these phrases popping up unsolicited throughout the day: "I am not good enough," or "I am not able to complete this task." These affirmations seem so normal to us now, and positive ones might make us feel uncomfortable. Remind yourself that you deserve to be compassionate towards yourself. Always look for ways to include positive thoughts even if it's difficult to find them.

Throughout this meditation, ensure that you are allowing yourself to believe and understand the statements fully. You can pull some of your favorite ones and repeat them every day, or you can write them down and keep notes around your house so that you stay positive. Look for creative ways to include these affirmations in your life, but most importantly practice the other breathing exercises.

Affirmations for Positivity

I am a strong independent person. I do not need to depend on anyone. I am able to take care of myself. I am worthy of everything that comes my way. I understand how to get the things that I want from life. I am completely aware of the things that I am in control of. I'm not afraid of the things that are outside of my control.

_____ **Melanie Johnson**

I am a capable human being who can achieve anything I set my mind to. I will not let the fear of failure hold me back. I understand that sometimes, failure is a part of the process.

I am aware of how to use my mistakes to improve as an individual. I do not need to depend on anybody else for my own happiness. I do not place blame on other individuals for my own mistakes.

I do not blame anyone else for the bad things that have come into my life.

I am aware of the way that other people might influence certain things in my life, but I am not going to blame them for these things.

I understand what I have to do to achieve the things that I want.

I am a motivated person. I am able to motivate myself to get things done.

_____

Melanie Johnson

I do not look for any outside sources of motivation.

I have the ability to self-reflect and motivate myself from within.

I will always honor myself and do what I can to look out for me.

I will always respect myself and the goals I set so I can achieve the things that

I want. I know how to set goals and my mindset to be a happier and healthier person.

I am somebody who is actively committed to living a better and healthier life. I am always going to look for methods to improve my life. I will always seek out the moments that make me happier.

I am dedicated to doing the right thing. I am focused on getting the things that

I want from this life because I know what I deserve.

I am not afraid of being an individual who is not going to get the things that I want.

I know exactly how to get the things that I desire the most. My ideas are clear, I have clear and realistic goals, I also have realistic expectations for the things that I will get from this life.

I do not hurt myself.

Once I do not achieve a goal.

I do not punish myself just because I don't get something that I wanted. I do not hurt myself because I am not happy with who I am. I only love myself. I love the person that I am. I use constant compassion to build myself up. I'm able to self-reflect in a healthy way.

I am aware of my flaws but I do not beat myself up over them.

I know the things that I need to work on. I understand my weaknesses, but I do not let these define me as somebody weak. I know how to change my life in order to get things that I want.

I will not let these weaknesses hold me back.

I am aware of these weaknesses and I am ever vigilant of working on them.

I understand my flaws and recognize that they make me a unique and interesting individual.

I have my own thought processes that are very important to the creativity and uniqueness that I exude.

I let go of all my negative feelings, and instead replace them with positive thoughts. I am able to self-reflect on my negative thoughts in a healthy way, and make sure that I turn them around.

I know how to seek out the positive and everything that comes my way. I am aware of the way that I can switch a negative perspective and turn it into a positive one. I choose to be positive every day. I understand what a privilege it is to be able to think within the full scope of your mind. I understand there will still be some days where I can't think positively, but I'm going to commit myself to always trying my best.

I let go of the negative thoughts and emotions of the past. I do not keep myself attached to the toxic mentality that has kept me chained back before. I embrace positivity, and I'm not afraid to be a happy person. I recognize that I am allowed to be happy. I am aware that it is okay for me to be positive. Just because other people aren't positive does not mean that I am not allowed to be.

I can be happy. I will be happy. I am happy. I am comfortable with the person that I am. I am happy and grateful for my body.

I understand that I could change things if I wanted to, but I am learning to accept me for me. I do not wish to be anybody else. I hope to change things for the better, but I still appreciate my unique characteristics. I admire other people, but I do not emulate them. I am myself. I am an individual. I have my own important character.

I am aware of all the things that I want to change about myself. I only have realistic expectations and look to change myself for the better. I am grateful for who I am. I am appreciative of the experiences that I have had because they have shaped me into the person I am today. I accept everything that has happened to me, because if not, then that would mean that I might not be the same person. I still have things to work on, but I am appreciative of the character that I have right now.

All the things that I have experienced have created the person that I am. I am thankful for these experiences because I love who I am, I am happy with the person that I have become. I do not want to know what might have happened if anything else had gone a different way. I'm accepting that this is the reality and I am not going to try to change it anymore.

I am only looking to build a better and brighter future. I am very aware of everything that I need to do in order to get the things that I want. I am powerful, and I am capable. I am able, and I am willing. I am ready, and I am excited. I am not afraid. I am not frightened; I am not going to let anything stop me. I'm always going to look for a way to improve my life. I am a happy person. Everyone around me knows that I am a happy person. My life matters and it has value.

I have value as an individual; my character has virtue and will share that with others. I am inspiring to myself and to the people that are around me. I am able to accomplish anything that I set my mind to. I permit myself to be positive, and to be happy. I know that being negative is not going to help me. I know that having a negative mindset is only going to hold me back.

I am aware of all the useful things that I do in this world. I am able to contribute to others and to my own life. I use positivity to get me through the most challenging moments in life. I am able to let go of any negative feelings that might come my way. I make the right decisions and use positivity to get me through. I have a high level of virtue.

I focus on healing my inner child, and I make sure that my choices have integrity. I look for ways to work past my negative thoughts. I know how to get to the root of thought. I know that my past experiences have created the person that I am today. I accept the things that have happened to me, but I do not let them define me. I create my own definitions.

I understand that my situation worked out exactly as it needs to be.

I understand that even though something might not be good now that there is a plan and I will be able to see positivity in the end. Even though not everything might happen for a reason, I can still find a reason for everything that has happened.

I use hope and optimism to expect the best.

I do not attach my feelings to situations, so I am not disappointed if things don't go the way I planned. I know that I will still be strong enough to push through. I can use positivity to make sure that I make it through any situation that comes my way.

I refuse to give up because I care about myself. I love who I am, and I'm always going to fight for the best.

_____

Melanie Johnson

Hypnosis and the Power of the Mind

Our minds are very strong tools in our lives. How we behave and react to situations is a result of our mental conditioning and thought process. For a person to transform a certain behavior, for instance, quitting smoking or kicking an addiction to electronic devices, the transformation must start in mind first. What we instill in our subconscious minds is want we portray outside. For instance, if you are overweight due to overeating or eating the wrong kinds of foods, there may be underlying issues to your behavior. To transform your behavior, you must begin by transforming your mind. By use of hypnosis, a person can transform their mind and achieve their desired change.

Using Hypnosis to Transform your Mind

The idea of hypnotherapy brings out reactions ranging from "cross-arm and wary in dismay" to "shocked in unadulterated amazement and surprise." There is no denying the supernatural quality encompassing spellbinding; it stays to puzzle individuals' psyches around the world.

As a result, we tend to live our lives amid a society in which the day to day rush of events doesn't leave us much time for thought and contemplation. This means that we are faced with making difficult choices in terms of dealing with our happiness and wellbeing.

Fortunately, this idea is a long way from a reality of true to life when you grasp spellbinding. In this way, we have a greatly improved idea. What about utilizing the incredible intensity of hypnotherapy rather than manufacturing a universe of a completely perfect world?

Since there is a persuading reason for hypnotherapy behind the cloak of wizardry and visual impairment, to fix our brains, bodies, and in the long run our universe.

As a general rule, trance has been utilized worldwide as an instrument for mending for in any event 4,000 years; however, science has just begun to exhume this entrancing riddle in most recent years. Their outcomes hugely affect our ability to change our thoughts and convictions, conduct, and practices, just as our recognition and reality to improve things.

In any case, most importantly, science has discovered a solid reality: entrancing is valid. What's more, on the off chance that you accept you've never had mesmerizing, accept again.

Hypnosis' characterizing practices are:

- *Increased suggestibility*. Making musings progressively open and responsive.
- *Improved creative thinking*. Creation in the eye of our psyches of striking, frequently illusory symbolism.

- *Without thinking, discernment.* Quieting the cognizant systems that create thoughts while improving passionate mindfulness.

These 3 characterizing highlights make spellbinding a particular and effective instrument for private transformation.

A large portion of the issues that unleash destruction on the globe today happen because we have significant mental wounds to which there has been no inclination.

We download information from the globe around us at lightning speed until we're around 9 years of age. During this minute, our subliminal feelings and practices are normally shaped — before we built up our balanced reasoning (got when our mind frames the prefrontal cortex).

In our childhood, for instance, someone can let us know, "you're ugly." At the time, our brains can't defend the likelihood that any individual who reveals to us this will have a poor day or experience the ill effects of their psychological wounds. Rather, our energetic, honest personalities accept, "goodness, I'm frightful." That works for "you're stunning" on a kinder note, just as some other great attestation.

We are importance making machines in this incredibly porous minute in our life. We quickly credit importance to them when certain events happen in our youthfulness. What produces our subliminal convictions are that allotted significance.

This is the place hypnotherapy comes in. Nothing fixes these significantly established enthusiastic wounds more rapidly than the hypnotherapy prescription. We have discovered that, in the condition of mesmerizing, we can get to and interface legitimately with these intuitive zones of our psyche—without our normal cognizant reasoning.

During trance, a trance inducer controls their patients back to their youth's zenith occasions. The patient can reassign centrality to them once recollections of the case are gotten to.

Reprogramming your Mind through Hypnosis

Your intuitive personality has an enormous impact in dealing with your background—from the sorts of sustenance you eat to the exercises you take each day, the income level you get, and even how you react to unpleasant conditions.

Your intuitive feelings and understandings manage all of it. In a nutshell, your subliminal personality resembles an airplane's auto-pilot work. Following a particular way has been pre-modified, and you cannot go astray from that course except if you initially change the customized guidelines.

The "intuitive" is your mind's part that works underneath your customary arousing cognizance level. At this moment, you are primarily utilizing your cognizant personality to peruse these expressions and retain their centrality. However, your subliminal personality works hectically in the background, engrossing, or dismissing information dependent on a present perspective on the globe around you. When you were a tyke, this present observation began to shape. Your intuitive personality drenches like wipe data with each experience.

While you were youthful, your consciousness rejected nothing since you had no prior perspectives that would negate what it saw. It simply recognized that it was genuine every one of the information you acquired during your initial puberty. You can almost certainly observe why this sometime down the road turns into an issue. Each time you were called by somebody stupid, useless, slow, apathetic, or more terrible, your subliminal personality put away the information for reference.

You may likewise have messages about your life potential or requirements relying upon your physical aptitudes, the shade of the skin, sex, or money related status. By the minute you were 7 or 8 years of age, you had a solid premise of religious on all the programming you viewed from people in your lives, network shows, and other natural impacts.

Since you are developed, you may simply dispose of the destructive or false messages you've consumed in your initial life. However, it isn't so basic. Keep in mind this information is put away underneath your cognizant awareness level. The main minute you understand this is the point at which it constrains your advancement in building up an actual existence that is adjusted, prosperous, and gainful.

Have you, at any point, endeavored to arrive at a target and consistently undermined yourself? Goading, right? It is fundamental to comprehend that regardless of what you do, you are not flawed or destined to come up short. You are bound to have some old, customized messages that contention with the new conditions that you need to make.

This is incredible news since it suggests that on the off chance that you first set aside the effort to reconstruct your intuitive personality, you can achieve pretty much anything! Before we discover how to reconstruct your psyche, it's fundamental to comprehend that the programming proceeds right up 'til today. You draw certain discoveries with each experience you have and store the messages that will direct your future conduct.

Procedures to Reprogram your Mind

There are numerous particular techniques to overwrite your psyche mind's constrained or hurtful messages.

You could work with every one of these methodologies simultaneously; however, on the off chance that you pick only a couple of procedures to start, it will be significantly more effective. Rather than skipping around and weakening your endeavors, you need to give them complete consideration. Keep in mind;

additional strategies can generally be consolidated after some time.

Impacts from the Environment around you

Have you, at any point, respected your psyche mind's effect on your setting? Keep in mind that your subliminal personality is always engrossing information and reaching determinations dependent on that information and framing convictions.

Envision what sorts of messages are being ingested into your psyche if your day by day condition is loaded up with cynicism and struggle. Your first meditation is to carefully limit from this time on the antagonism to which you are oppressed. Except if you thoroughly need to watch the news and avoid investing a lot of energy with' lethal' people.

Rather, search for helpful information to peruse and watch, and burn through the vast majority of your minute with people who are sure and effective. You will locate that all the more reassuring messages are retained into your brain after some time, which will change how you see yourself and your potential.

Representation

Your subliminal personality responds well to pictures. Representation is an amazing method to utilize ideal, incredible pictures to program your brain. Attempt to picture advantageous scenes that element you and your background for 10–15 minutes every day.

Here are a few things you should envision:

- Fulfilling connections
- Passionate work
- An exquisite home extraordinary excursion

Whatever else you need to bring into your lives. As you do this always, you wind up redrawing the unfavorable pictures put away from your past encounters, concerns, concerns, and questions. Make sure to emanate incredible, positive emotions as you picture these excellent things in your brain to expand the quality of representation further. Permit love, satisfaction, appreciation, and harmony to move through you as though you genuinely had these encounters.

The message will be consumed by your subliminal personality, as though it were real! This is the genuine excellence of perception—the expert to sidestep confining messages and focuses on beautiful pictures that are altogether retained into your subliminal to replay later.

Affirmations

Affirmations are another practical method to place positive messages into your intuitive.

On the off chance that you observe a couple of straightforward standards, they work best:

- *Positively word them in the current state.* Declare "I'm certain and fruitful" rather than "I will be sure and effective," because are concentrating on a future condition doesn't compute with your intuitive personality — it just comprehends this time. Utilize helpful articulations too. Saying "I am not a disappointment" is determined as "I am a disappointment" since it is incomprehensible for your intuitive to process negative things.

- *Call for the proper feelings.* Saying "I am rich" while feeling poor just sends your subliminal clashing messages. Whatever words you state right now, attempt to feel the sentiments because your intuitive will be bound to think it.

- *Repeat, reiteration, redundancy.* On the off chance that you simply state it on more than one occasion, certifications don't work. The decent thing about this is you can reveal to yourself attestations so that they can accommodate your routine flawlessly.

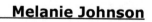

Self-Hypnosis for Peaceful Sleep

Who can pursue deep-sleep self-hypnosis?

Anyone who has an active lifestyle but finds their sleep pattern disturbed can seek this treatment.

Mostly, this applies to the working individuals in any field.

For children this relaxation technique isn't recommended.

Locate an agreeable, calm spot to sit or rest

Take your place

You can do this practice sitting or lying down

Stay in completely relaxed manner

Don't do anything immediately

Ground yourself first

Just sit or lie down completely relaxed for a few minutes

Get into a comfortable position

Keep your back straight

Ensure that your shoulders are also straight

Your back and neck should be in a straight line

Now, gently close your eyes

Notice if there is tension anywhere in your body

If you feel any part tense, release the tension

Adjust your body to release the pressure

Start breathing normally

Breathe in slowly

Let the air enter through your nostrils

Fill your lungs with the air

Hold your breath for a few moments

Now, release the breath slowly through your mouth

Take a deep breath

And hold it

Now slowly exhale

Breathe in deeply

Feel the calm energy filling you

Hold your breath

And slowly release

Every exhalation takes away stress and negativity

Don't hurry up

Take your time to relax

Again, breathe in

Hold

And breathe out

You are feeling good, there is nothing disturbing you

You are calm and relaxed now

1 - Imagine the routine scenarios at home that you
experience every day

Notice minute things such as color of the wall paintings,
night shade etc.

Imagine as many details as you can

2 - Now imagine yourself changing into your nightwear
before going to bed

While you are undressing

Let your connection to the current day go

All the friendly or official talks

Each one of the memories, casual talks and gossips

Must be discarded alongside any worries

Consider the clothing you are wearing as the stress

And get it mentally off bit by bit

Feel the tension getting away

Feel yourself comfortable, calm and relaxed

3 - Now visualize your usual night rituals

Such as taking a shower, brushing your teeth, lighting
incense sticks and so on

Meanwhile, do not speak much

Focus on the task in hand

You can envision that each stroke of your toothbrush is

getting rid of the dirt (stress)

Washing your negative thoughts

And lightening clearing your head of worries

Imagine watching yourself in third person calmly

When you feel it working, at that point proceed onward

to the subsequent stage

4 - Now imagine yourself getting into bed

And pull the sheets over yourself

If you do not use sheets, then think about an air-

blanket which is acting as your shield

And protecting yourself from negative thoughts and

influences

Consider that these sheets are your protectors from

unsettling influences and diversions

They shield you from emotions that you would prefer

not to contact you while you rest

Focus and think of it as your safe haven

Where you would not want your negative experiences

and emotions to come

Melanie Johnson

When you have a sense of safety

Feel safe and quiet

Proceed onward to the next stage

5 - Now imagine how you turn off the lights

Envision the darkness of the room enveloping your
issues and anxieties

and indicating them to stay away for this night

They can be tackled the next day

As you flick the turn off

You see a turn getting flicked off in your mind

That relinquishes everything without exception
undesirable

And gives you a chance to float to rest

Honestly do everything you can

And envision that switch being flipped inside your
psyche

And once you have done that

Proceed onward to the subsequent stage

6 - Now envision yourself, lying calmly in bed

Resting cheerfully, profoundly

And possibly longing for awesome things

Before floating into a profound, non-imagining rest

Simply watch yourself dozing significantly and
profoundly and flawlessly
And as you watch that
Ponder internally:
"I simply realize that will occur"
And truly get a definite feeling of realizing
That you will be resting that way very soon
Accept that you are resting better
Simply realize that you are resting better
Watch yourself resting euphorically
And after that proceed onward to the last step
7 - Bring yourself up and out of spellbinding
By squirming your fingers and toes
Taking a full breath
Opening your eyes

This relaxation technique should be repeated at least for
one week without any gap. At that point after you have
rehearsed it in your self-hypnotizing session. Practice
that tirelessly and as frequently as you can, and it'll
begin to have an extremely brilliant impact.

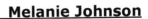

Melanie Johnson

Melanie Johnson

Script 1

Lie flat on your back and feel the sensations on your body for a while. Spread your hands and feet comfortably to make sure you are fully relaxed.

Now I want you to focus your attention on your breath.

I want you to breathe in deeply and fill the bottom of your lungs, causing the lower belly to rise. Hold your breath for a few seconds and slowly release the air while feeling your lower belly drop. Make sure you have emptied every drop of air from your lungs.

Start again by noticing how fresh the air is as you breathe in. Pay attention to filling your lower lungs with air as you feel your stomach rise again. Make sure you have filled your lungs with air that you cannot take in more.

Pause for a few seconds and let go of the air slowly. Repeat this process seven times. Each time, imagine your body relaxing and letting go of all the tension you have.

Let it all fade away as sand washed off by water.

Now, try to feel every bit of your body. Notice any points of tension and just make a note of them. I want you to start relaxing your muscles from the top of your head to your toes.

Tense the crown of your head and release the tension, pushing it to the left side of the head.

Tense the left side of your head and release any tension left while pushing it to the right side of the head. Do the same for the right side of the head and push the pressure to the back of the head.

Now, bring your attention to your forehead. Tense your forehead and do away with any tense sensation. If there are still traces of tension, move to the left and right eyebrow.

Each time, make sure you tense each part and release the pressure, pushing whatever residual tension left to the next part of the body.

Do this twice since it is a crucial area of stress. From your eyebrows, drop down to your nose and tense it making sure to release the tension after a few seconds. Now go to the jaw region and do the same.

Imagine all your tension accumulated at the jaw. Move it down to your neck through your throat. This time too, tense your neck and release the tension twice. When done, you are free to move to your chest region.

From the chest region, repeat the same process, covering each part systematically and not neglecting any region. When you encounter an area with a lot of tension, tense it and release it twice then progress to the other part.

After completing the cycle of the chest and stomach region, transfer your attention to your upper back. Feel any tension present on your left scapula. Your scapula is the bone that is present on the upper back.

Tense it and release the tension after a few seconds. Transfer the tension to the right scapula and tense it as well. Release the tension each time, making sure to transfer the pressure left to the next part of the body.

Now continue with the process until you reach your lower back. Make sure to release all the tension or carry the residual to the next part.

Now, bring all your tension to the tip of your spine, close to the neck, and imagine it sliding down to join both scapulae and connecting to the shoulders.

Focus on the fingers from the left hand now. Relax and stretch your hand. Tense the muscles in your hand and transfer to your wrist any remaining tension.

Add tension then relax, moving to your forearm the remaining tension. Add tension, then relax, and then transfer to your upper arm any remaining tension.

Tense, relax, and shift to your shoulder any remaining tension. Repeat the same process for the right hand.

When you bring the final tension to your left shoulder, slide both accumulated tensions down to the spine and through the scapulae to the hips.

Tense the hips and relax. Imagine the tension left whirling around in a circle, just disbanding itself disappearing.

Tense the hips and relax them again. Now, move any tension left in the opposite direction and think of it being washed away by a calming feeling.

Move any residual tension to the thighs. Tense both of them simultaneously and relax. Carry any residual tension to the knees.

Tense both of them and relax. Make sure to keep conscious of the moving tension to ensure the areas are free of tension.

Move down to the shins, tensing them and relaxing them simultaneously after a few seconds.

Carry any residual tension to the calves. Tense them and relax them twice. This is a significant area of tension. Pay close attention to it as you transfer any residual tension to the ankles. Tense and relax the ankles twice as well. Move to the heels and do the same.

Tense and relax them foot by foot. Release all the tension and transfer any left tension to the toes. Imagine all the tension oozing out from the tips of your toes and flowing out of your body. You now feel relaxed and ready to encounter the next journey to sleep.

Now with your completely relaxed body lying still on the bed, feel your body getting lighter and lighter. You can envision yourself floating up and heading for the clouds.

You want to go and lay on the cushions of the clouds. Your body, mind, and spirit is calm. You are now in the midst of heavy cushiony clouds. You can feel them comfortably rubbing on your skin as you drift into more cloud comfort.

They just keep coming and ones that are more comfortable keep showing up. You can also feel a slight gentle breeze drift you away. You are relaxed.

Now imagine yourself lying still in a drifting boat that keeps rowing from side to side in a slow-moving river. The clouds are still your cushion and it is the most comfortable thing you have ever experienced.

You are not worried where the river is flowing to; you are just drifting off with it, letting the rowing and the comfort of the cloud blanket be the center of your attention. You are in a safe environment. Anywhere you go is a familiar place. You can always find your way back home.

Look at the sides of the boat. Look how beautiful the trees are on each side, leaning a bit closer to the river. Notice how they form a protective canopy around you, protecting you from the sun and strong winds. It is refreshing and calm—just the right thing for you.

The birds are chirping with lulling songs. You like the song. You like the place. There are rays of sunshine peering through cracks from the canopy, giving you a warm feeling. The boat is still rowing.

The comfort of the clouds still engulfs you. There is no concept of time in this space as well. Time is entirely still. Your only concern is the relaxed feeling that has taken over your body. You can feel the sounds of the river flowing; it is so gentle and peaceful yet confident.

This makes you feel stress-free and calm. You do not have any care in the world.

Take two last deep breaths. The purpose is to put your body into more profound relaxation as you prepare to drift into deep sleep. Feel yourself sink further into your bed as you drift off into deep sleep. You are at peace and safe.

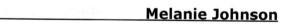

Melanie Johnson

Script 2

Begin in a comfortable position. Lie on your back with your hands at your sides or in your thighs. You have permission to switch positions at any moment to ensure maximum comfort, but for now, begin by lying comfortably on your back.

Do a quick mental scan on your body for any areas with tension. Take this time note, fully, how your body feels. In this session, your focus will be releasing all types of tension in your body and silencing the mind.

As soon as your mind is blank and free from anger and anxiety, you will easily find yourself engulfed by peaceful sleep.

Exhale slowly, expelling any tension.

You might be thinking about what you accomplished today and what you will need to accomplish tomorrow.

Maybe you are worried about a specific situation or individual. Perhaps you are concerned about the circumstances which are surrounding you at any given moment. Ideally, you would be able to identify what is affecting you.

To achieve relaxation and eventually sleep, you should erase everything from your mind so that tomorrow you will be relaxed, alert, and able to handle your responsibilities with a positive mentality.

Take some time to ponder on what you usually do before you sleep. For the next few minutes, do any fretting or pondering you decide on. You should now erase everything from your mind. Your focus should not be on anything else at this moment other than clearing your mind.

Take this moment to take into full account how your body feels.

Where is all the pent-up tension stored today? Focus all your energy on the area of your body that is experiencing the most tension. Focus all your energy on the smallest point of tension. Take a deep breath in and surround the tension, and as you exhale that breath, release all the tension with a sigh of relief.

Pay attention to the area in your body that is the most relaxed. Feel the relaxation build up with every breath you take. Let the feeling of relaxation explore your body further and further.

As you feel the sleep oozing into your system, feel your mind go deeper and deeper into the calm sensation.

For the following minutes, you may decide to focus on counting down as you breathe, and become more and more relaxed with each breath you take or as you continue counting. Focus your energy and attention on the number one and breathe calmly.

As you breathe, take your time to count from one, slowly getting to ten as you become calmer and your body more relaxed. As you let go, you need to allow yourself to drown in your relaxation and drift into a deep, refreshing slumber.

Continue breathing and mindfully count with me.

One, continue focusing on the number one as you breathe.

Two, you can feel yourself progressively sink into relaxation. The deeper you go, the calmer you get. Wallow in the peace.

Three, allow all the tension and negativity to escape your body. Let rest and relaxation fill your entire being. Concentrate on your breathing and the numbers.

Picture the number four as you sink deeper into relaxation. You can feel the relaxation move throughout your body, from your feet all the way to your arms. You feel your body becomes heavier and more substantial due to relaxation.

Focus all your remaining energy on the number five.

Allow your body and mind to sink deeper and deeper.

Six, you are experiencing intense relaxation.

Seven, accept the calmness that is embracing your
body and mind.

Eight, peaceful and intense relaxation.

Nine now allow your mind to sink more in-depth with a
lack of direction.

Ten, relaxation is flowing everywhere.

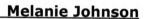

Melanie Johnson

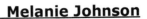

Melanie Johnson

Melanie Johnson